The Monster in Mykie

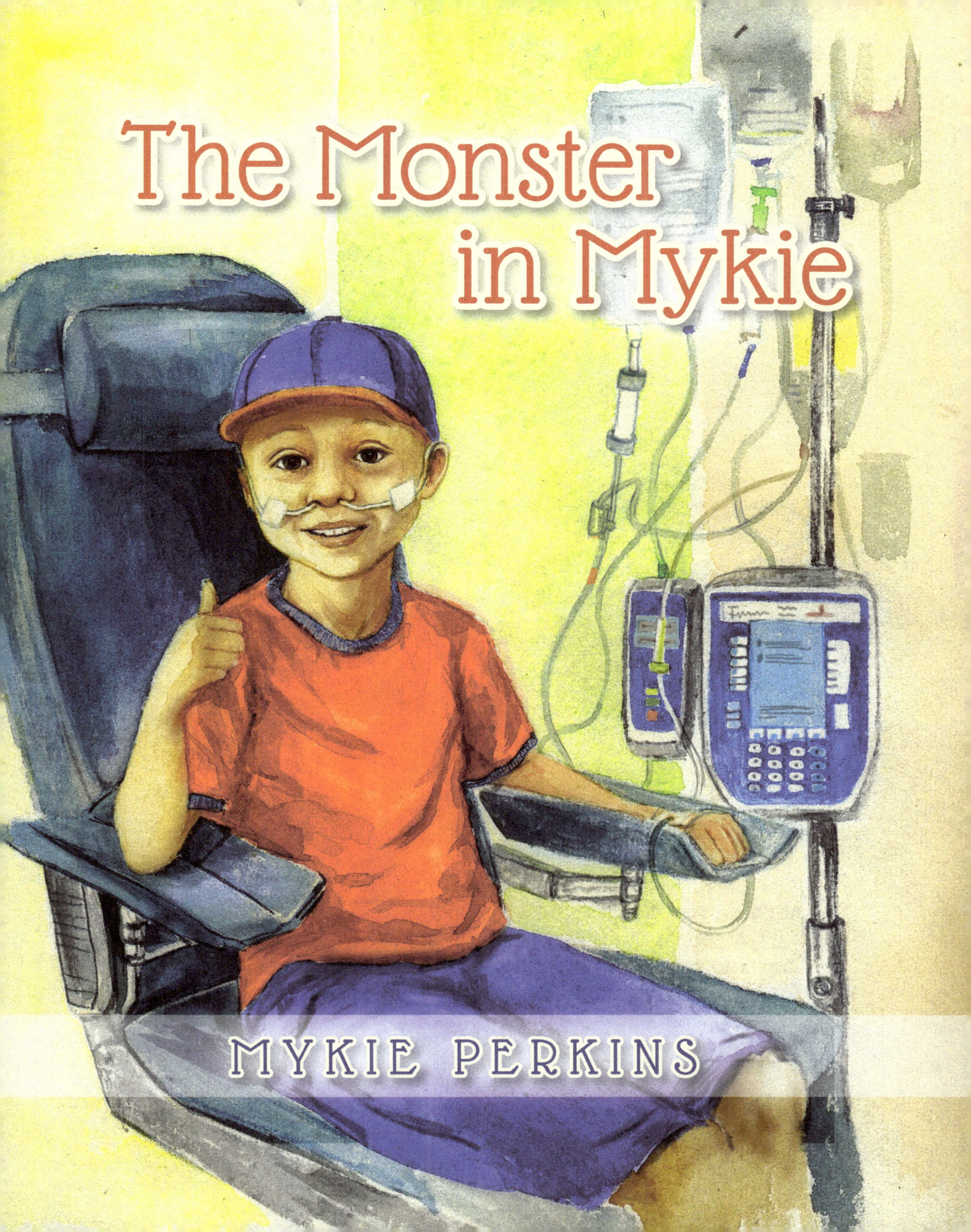

MYKIE PERKINS

ISBN: 978-1-9162194-1-0

The Monster Series
Published by Tiny Angel Press LTD.
Layout Design: Nonon Tech & Design

ACKNOWLEDGMENTS

Mum Dad and brother Tyler for encouraging and supporting me.
Donia Youssef for giving me the opportunity to raise awareness of childhood cancer.
All the children who have won the fight, continue to fight or gained their angel wings we are all warriors!

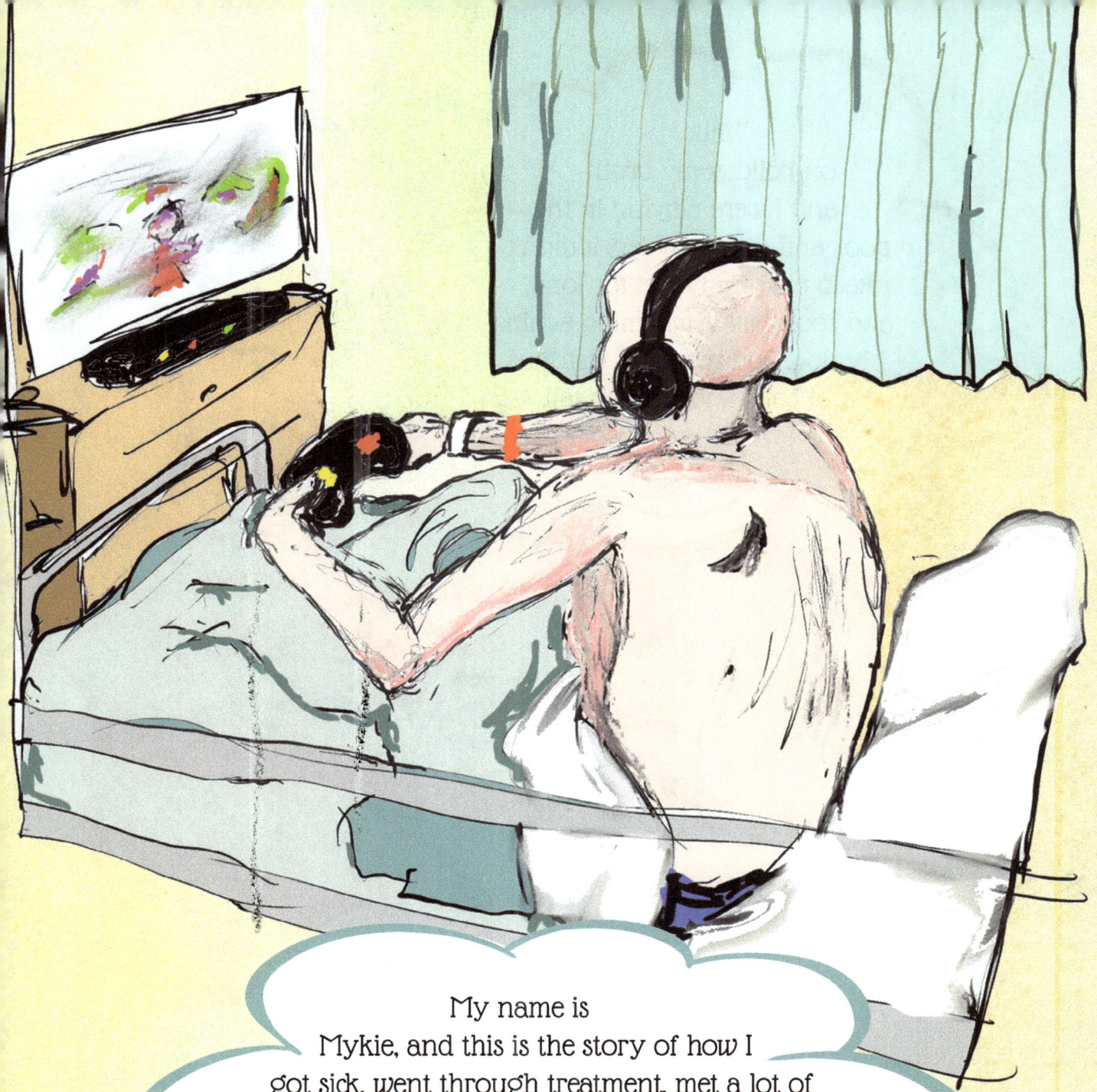

My name is
Mykie, and this is the story of how I
got sick, went through treatment, met a lot of
wonderful people, and finally, got better again!
Like most boys, I like Football, play station and I
really want to be a pilot when I am older.

While on holiday, my brother and I were playing in the pool, and I hurt my leg. It didn't keep me off my feet for long, and soon I was swimming again. My dog, Buddy, would watch us and bark and wag his tail.

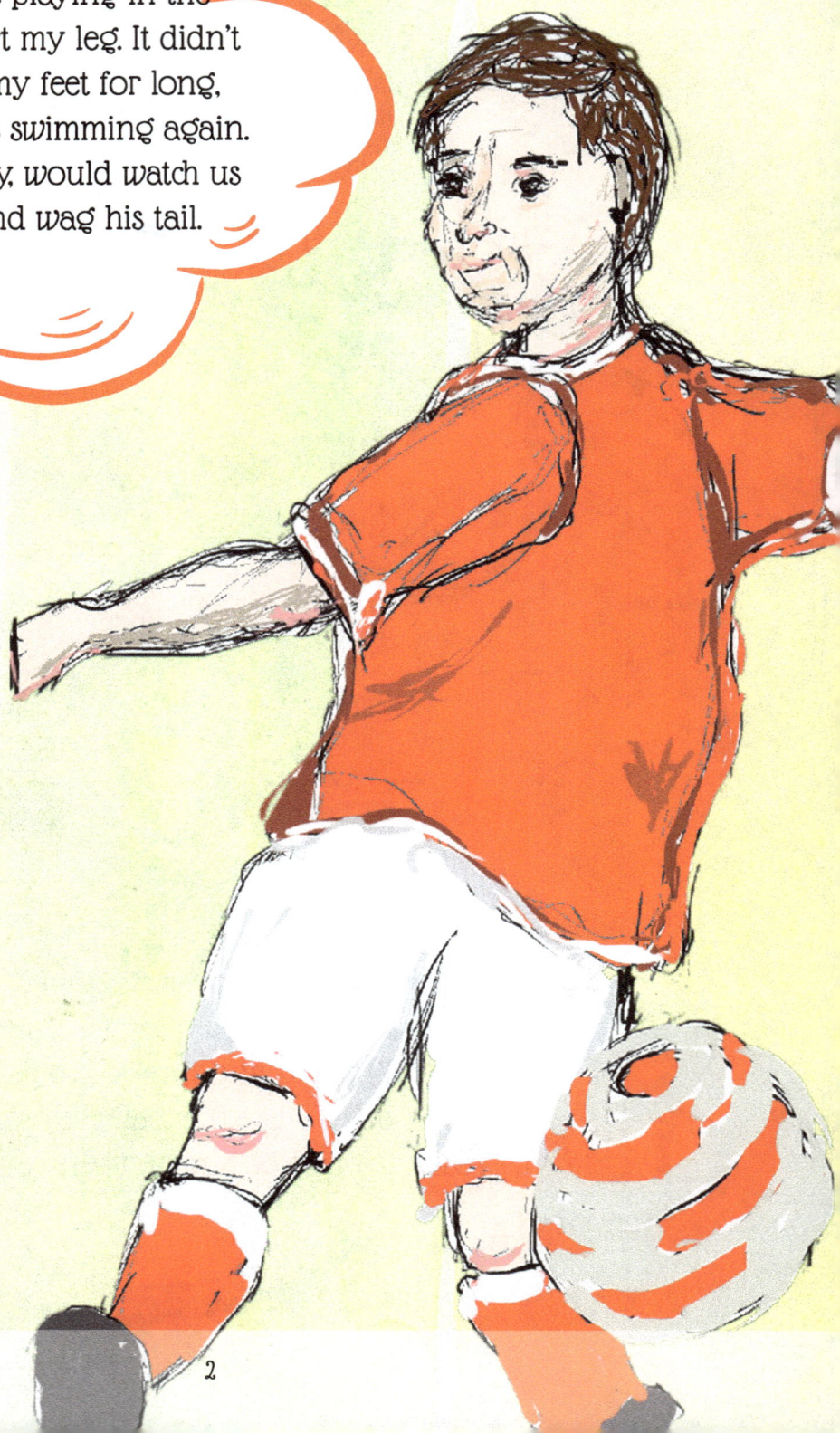

2

Over the
next few weeks, my leg began hurting
more at night; there was also a big lump. I named
him Larry–Larry the Lump!
Mum and dad were worried, so we went to the hospital to check my leg. After an X-ray, the doctor said I
had broken my leg, which really shocked me
as I was still walking.

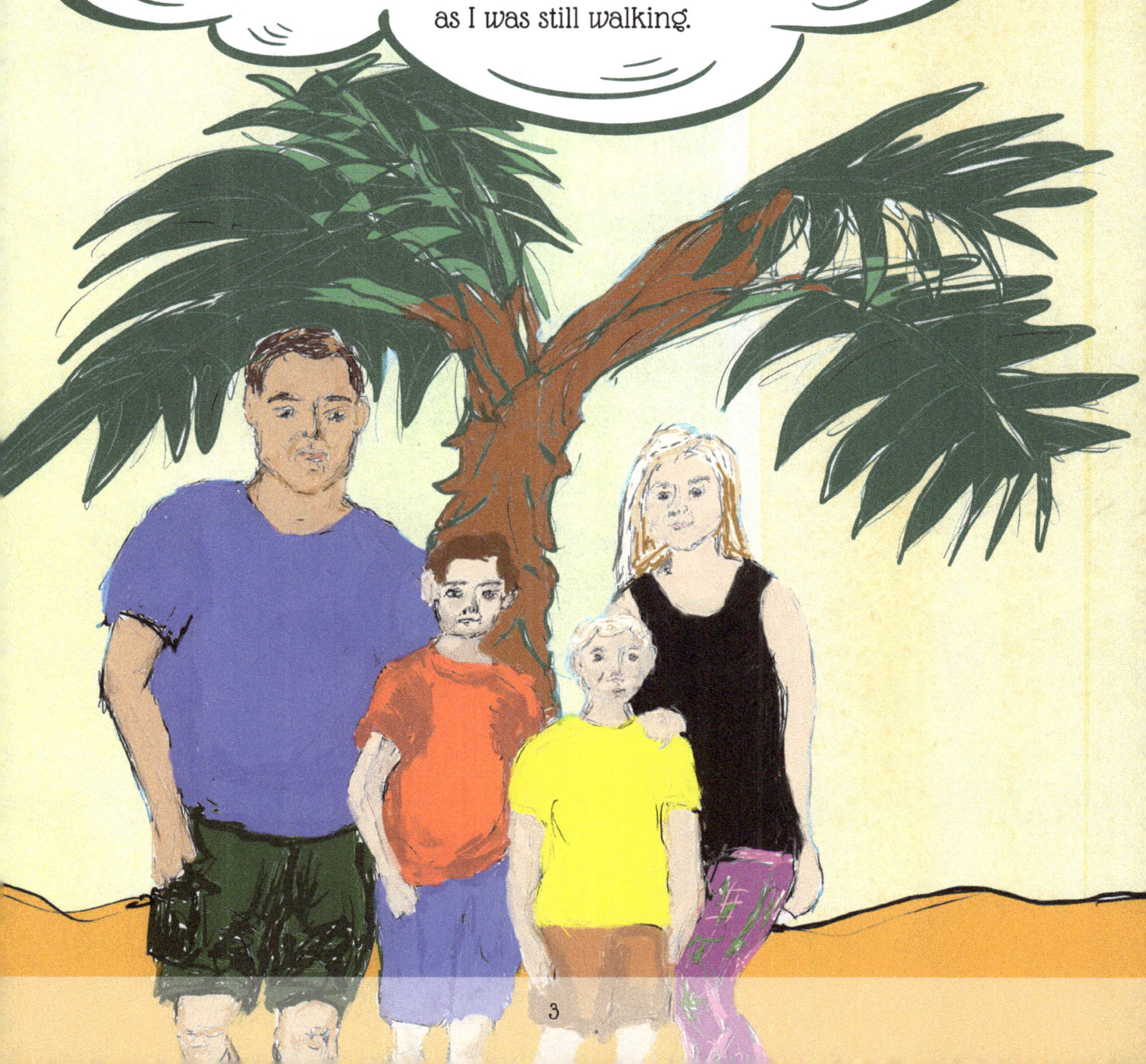

3

So, I went home, thinking I would need a cast and crutches, but two days later, the hospital called me back; they had reviewed my X-ray and said my leg was not broken, but instead, I had a tumor in my bone. The doctors told me and my parents that I had something called Ewing's sarcoma, which is a tumor that grows in the bones or tissues around the bones.

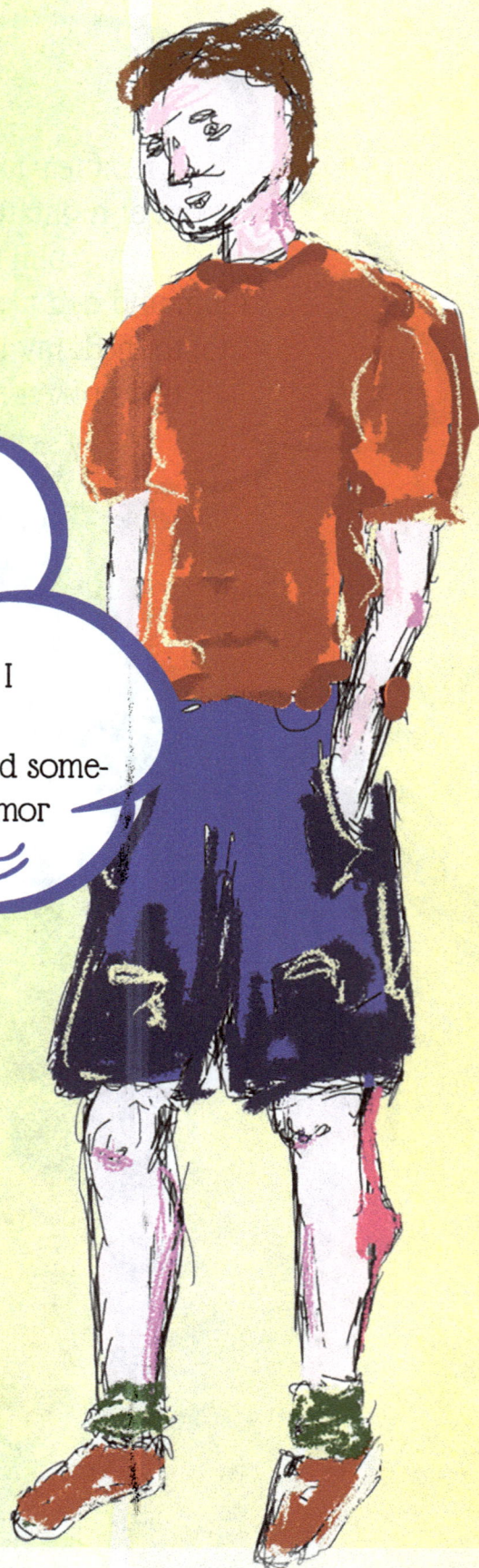

So, I went
to a bone specialist hospital. They
put me to sleep and took a sample of the
tumor. I woke up very hungry and ate a love-
ly chicken dinner. There was also a really nice
nurse who looked after me named Ollie. He
made me laugh so much.

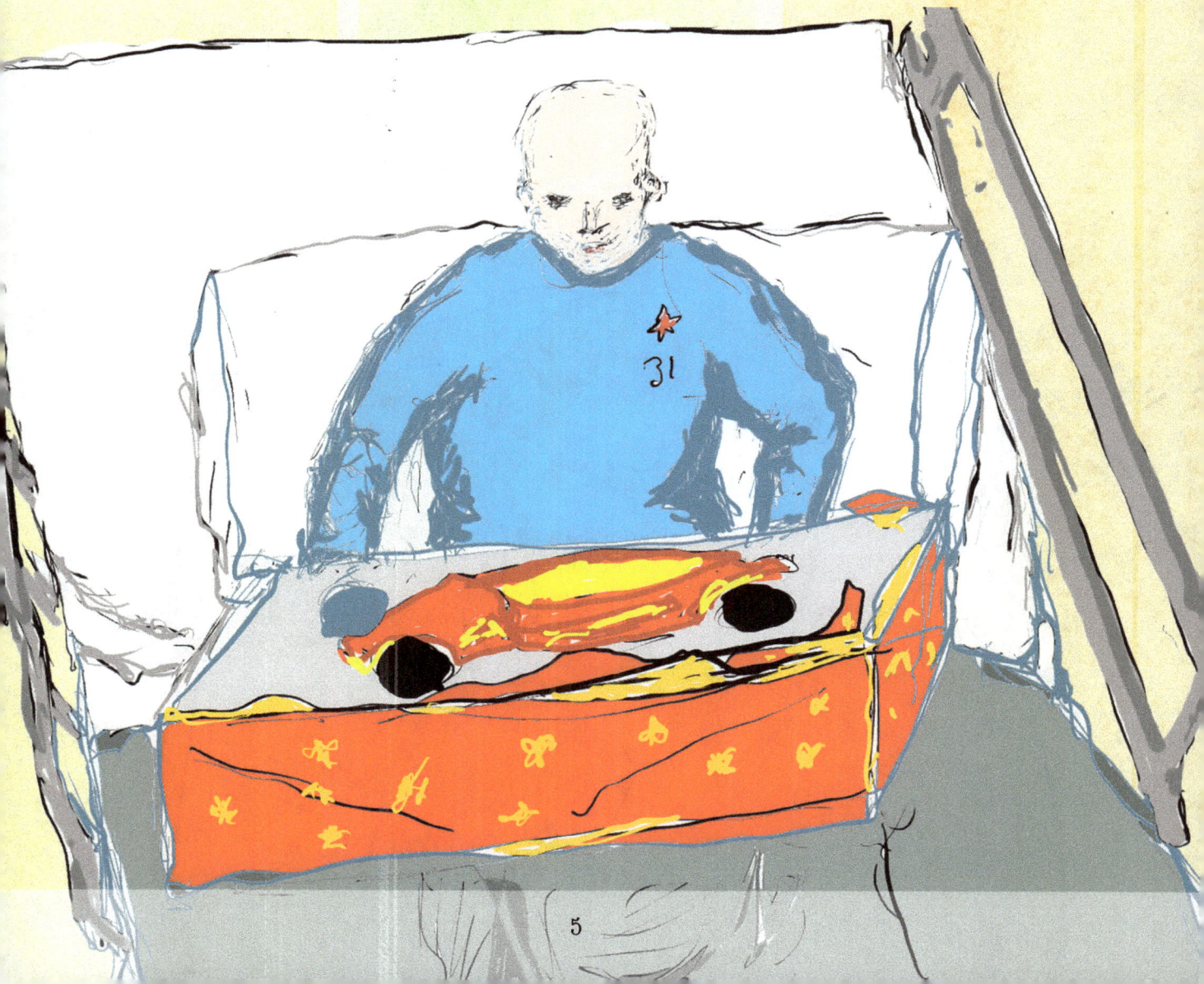

I also met
a new friend, who really, really
helped me. Her name was Katie, and she
was only twelve years old, but she'd already
been through a lot. She had a brain tumor, but
always had a smile on her face and told me
all sorts of things about what to expect.

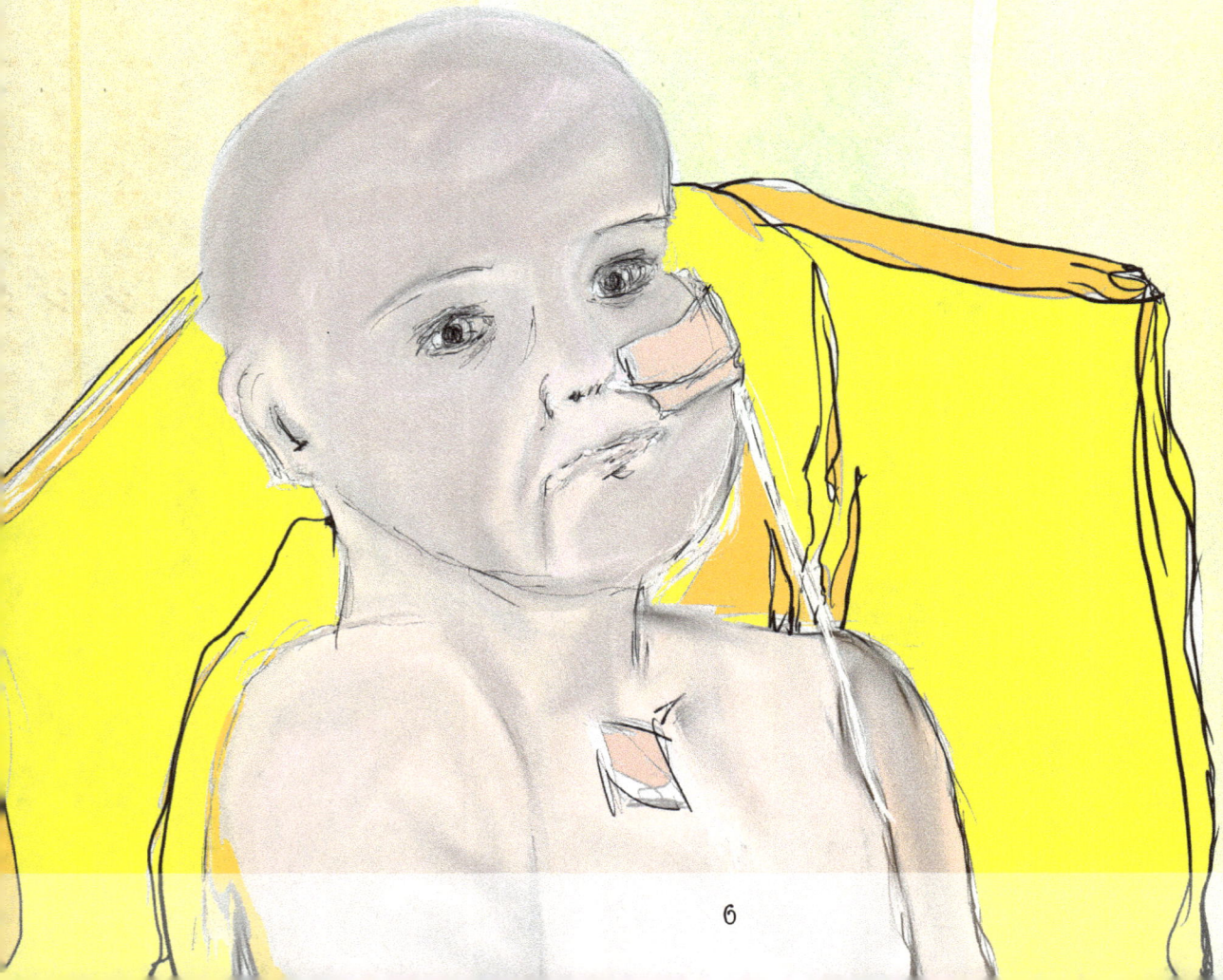

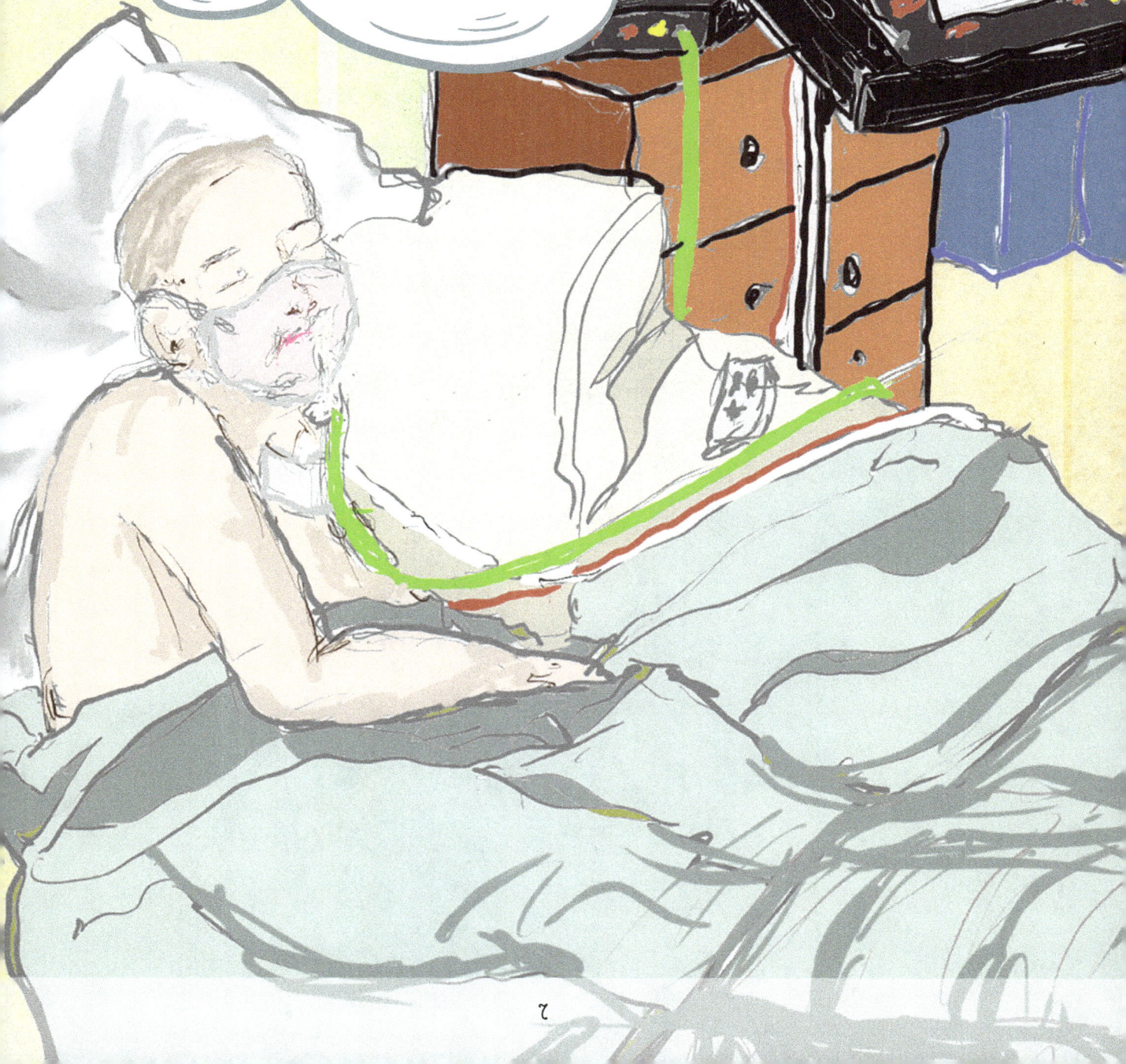

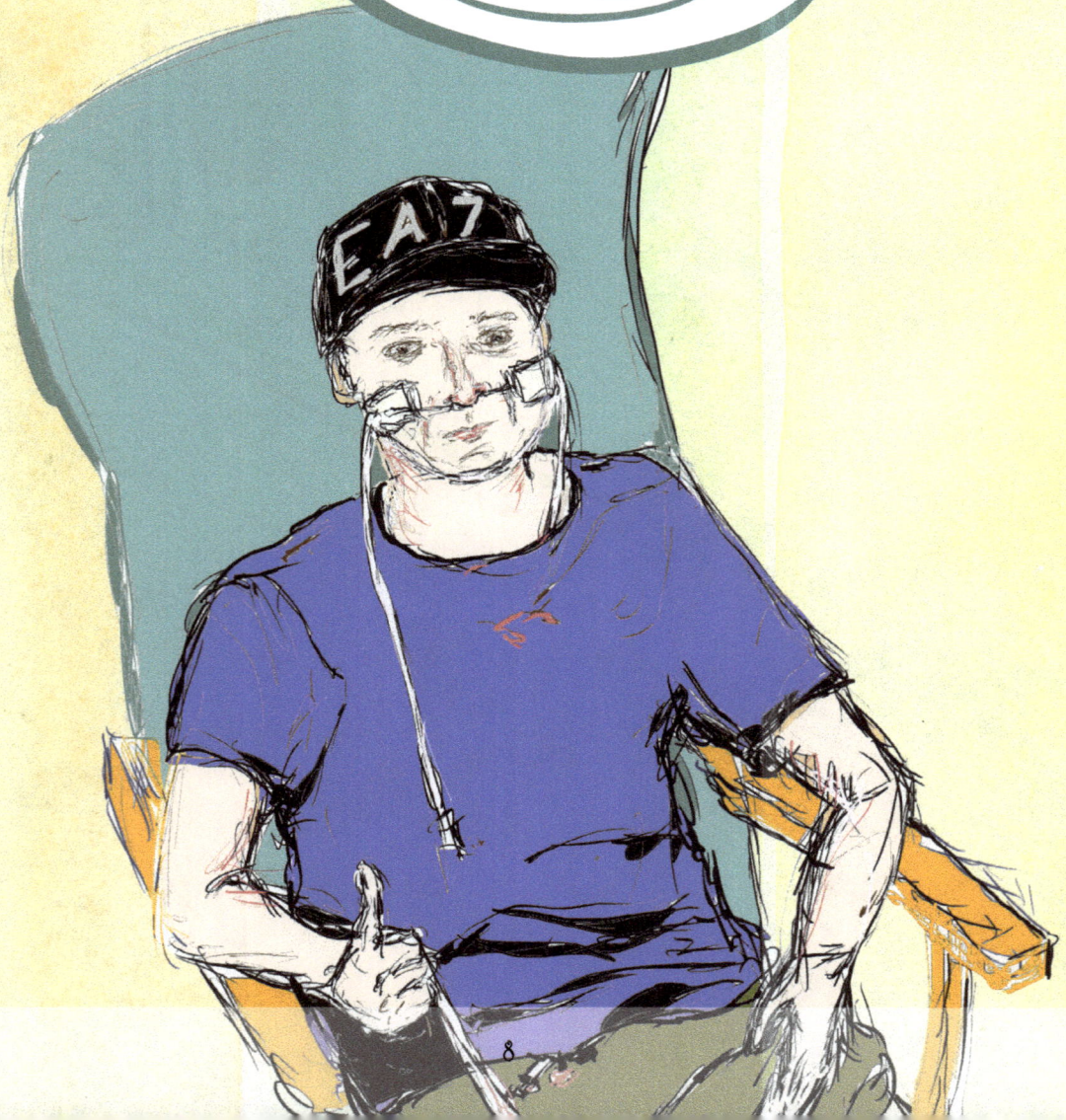

I spent eight days in Stanmore hospital. My leg was really sore, and I couldn't walk, but with lots of physical therapy, I was allowed to go home in a wheelchair. They also gave me a pair of crutches for when I wanted to walk around.

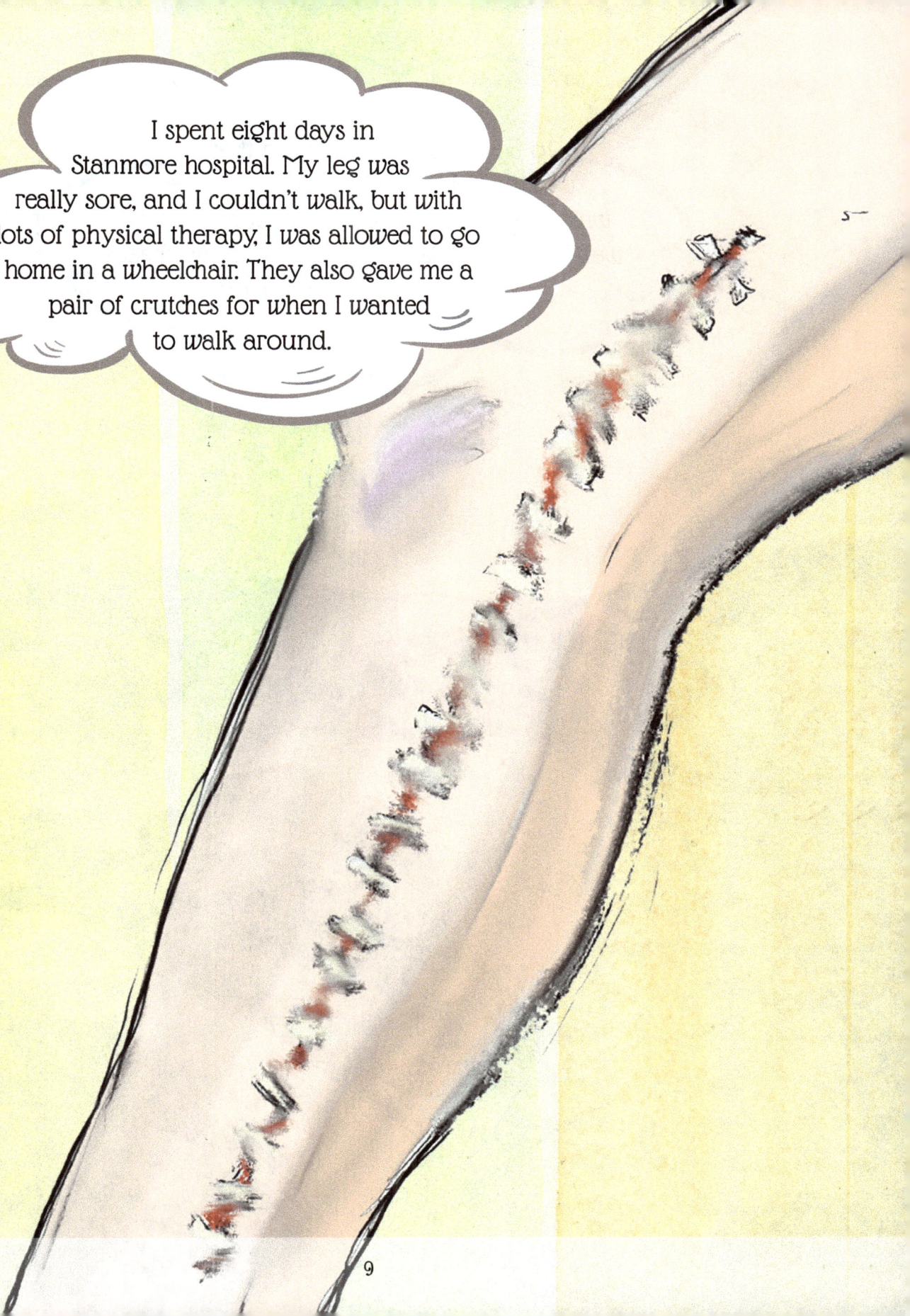

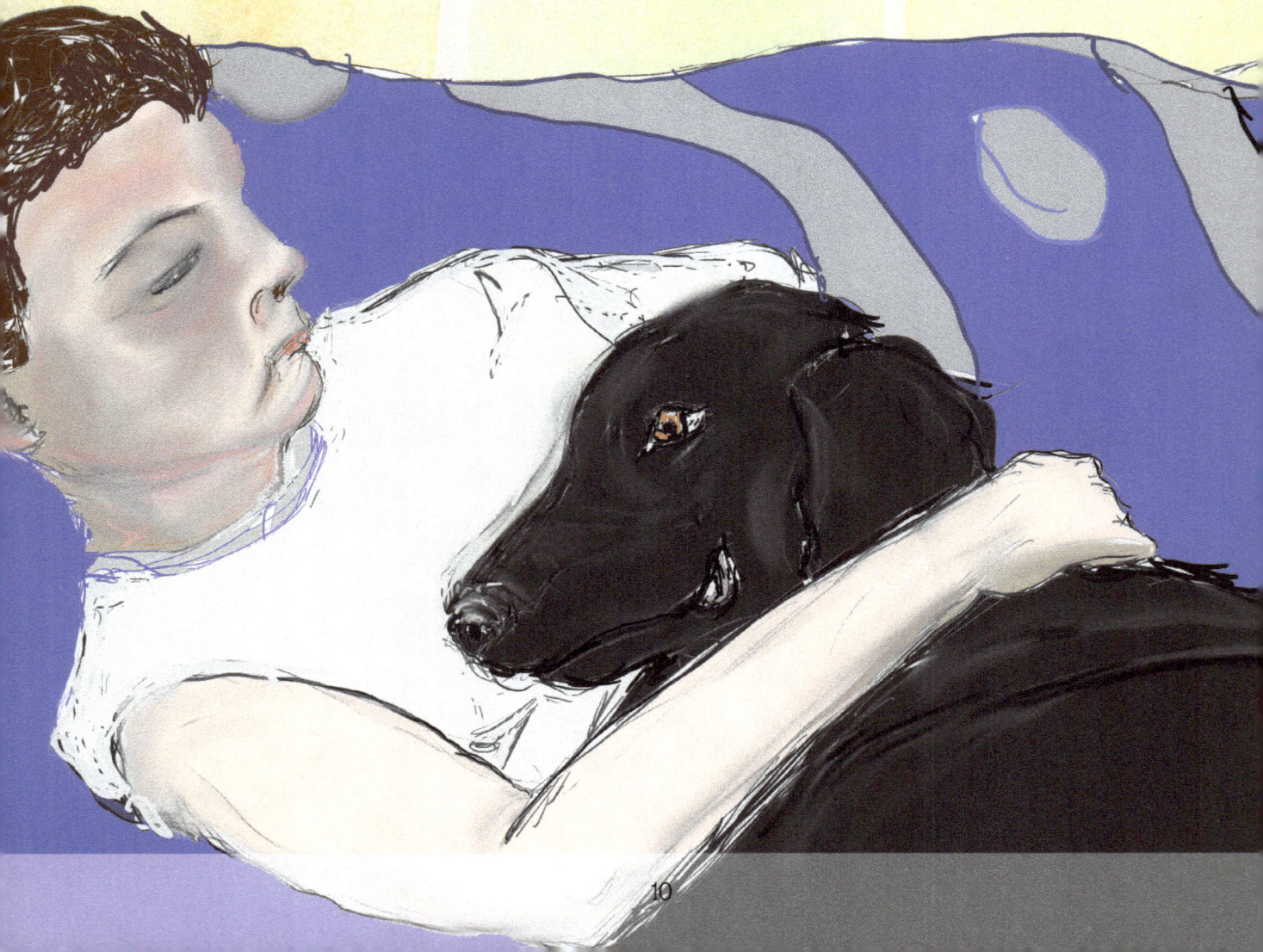

I was glad
to be home, but a little sad that I
was in a wheelchair. I was cancer-free,
which made me so happy. And Buddy would
wag his tail and lay with me, licking my cheeks
and keeping me company.

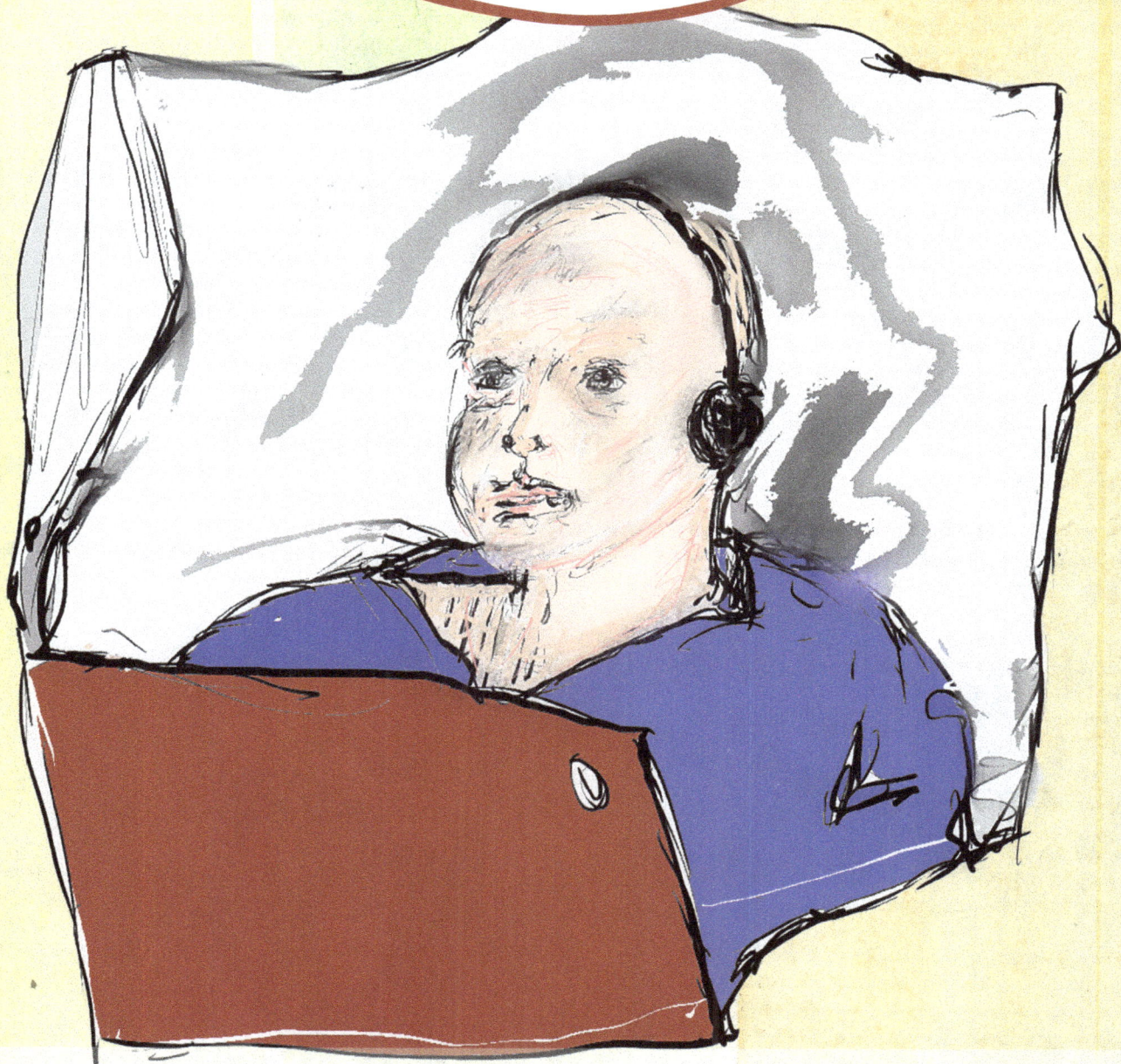

I had regular scans and tests at the hospital, and I also took a special medicine called Zoledronic acid once a month. This helped to heal the bone and prevent my cancer from coming back.

After my surgery, I had to have five more cycles of chemo, but they were not as intense and were not as hard on my body.

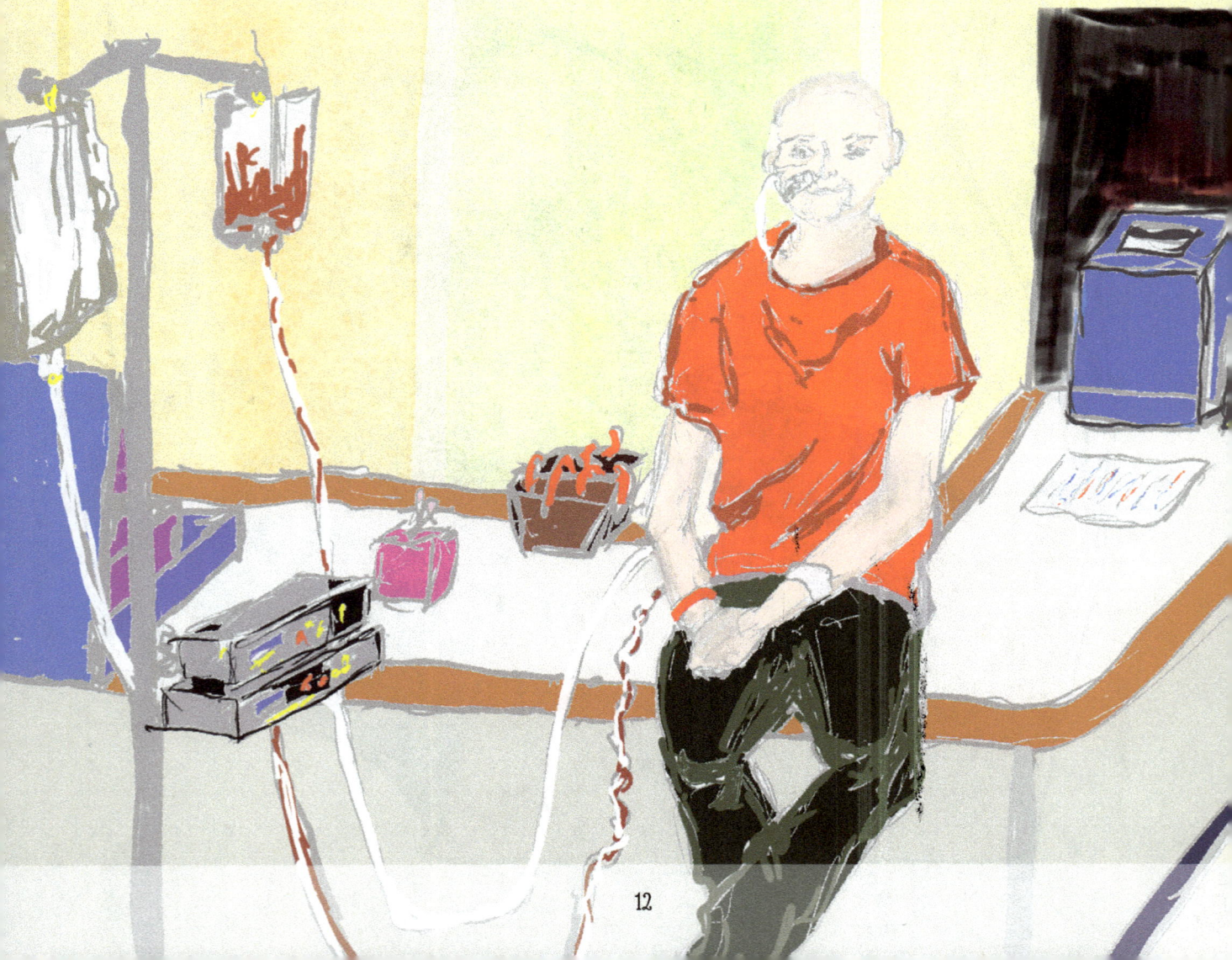

I enjoyed going up to the hospital every month because I got to see the nurses and the friends I had made.

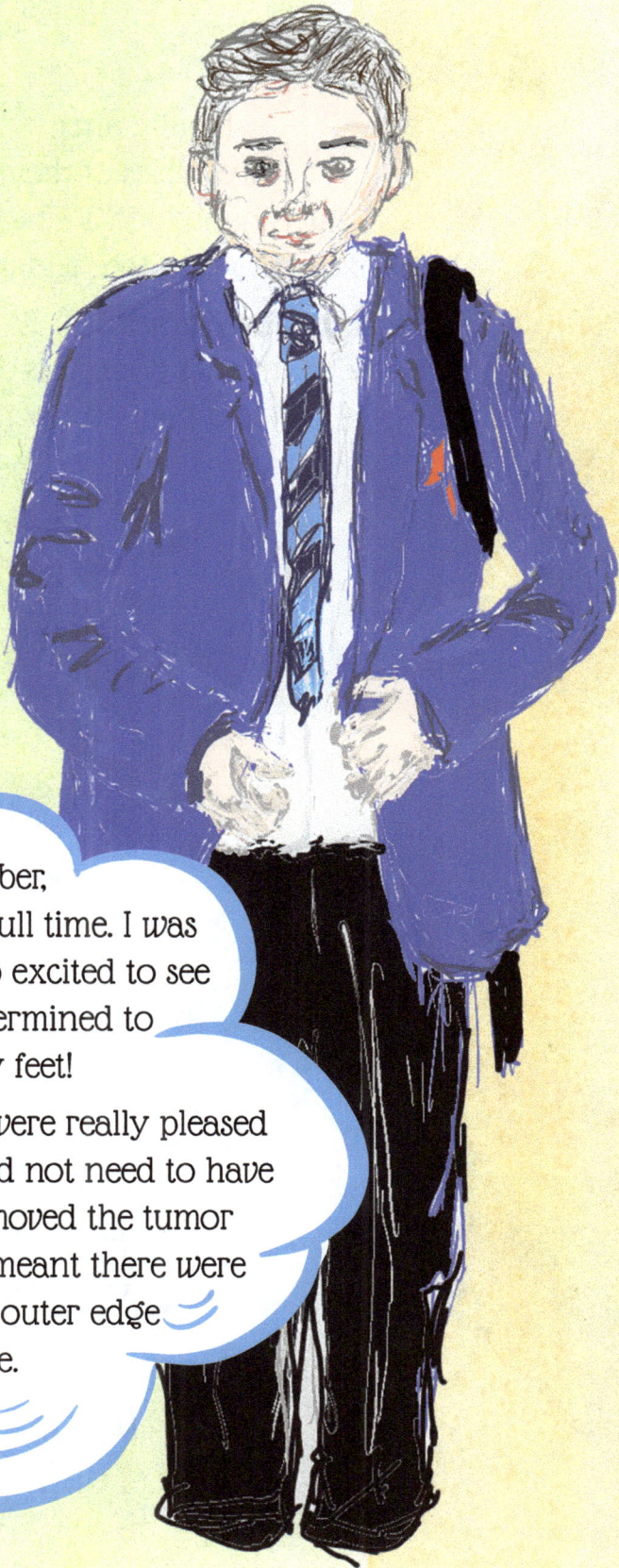

In September,
I went back to school full time. I was
quite nervous but also excited to see
my friends and determined to
get back on my feet!

The doctors told us they were really pleased
with my progress, and I did not need to have
radiotherapy as they removed the tumor
with clear margins, which meant there were
no cancer cells at the outer edge
of the tissue.

Finally, after
five cycles of chemo,
I was happy for it all to be over.
I was excited to ring the "end of treatment" bell.

Ring this bell three times well. Its time to clearly say
my treatment's done, this course is run,
and I am on my way!

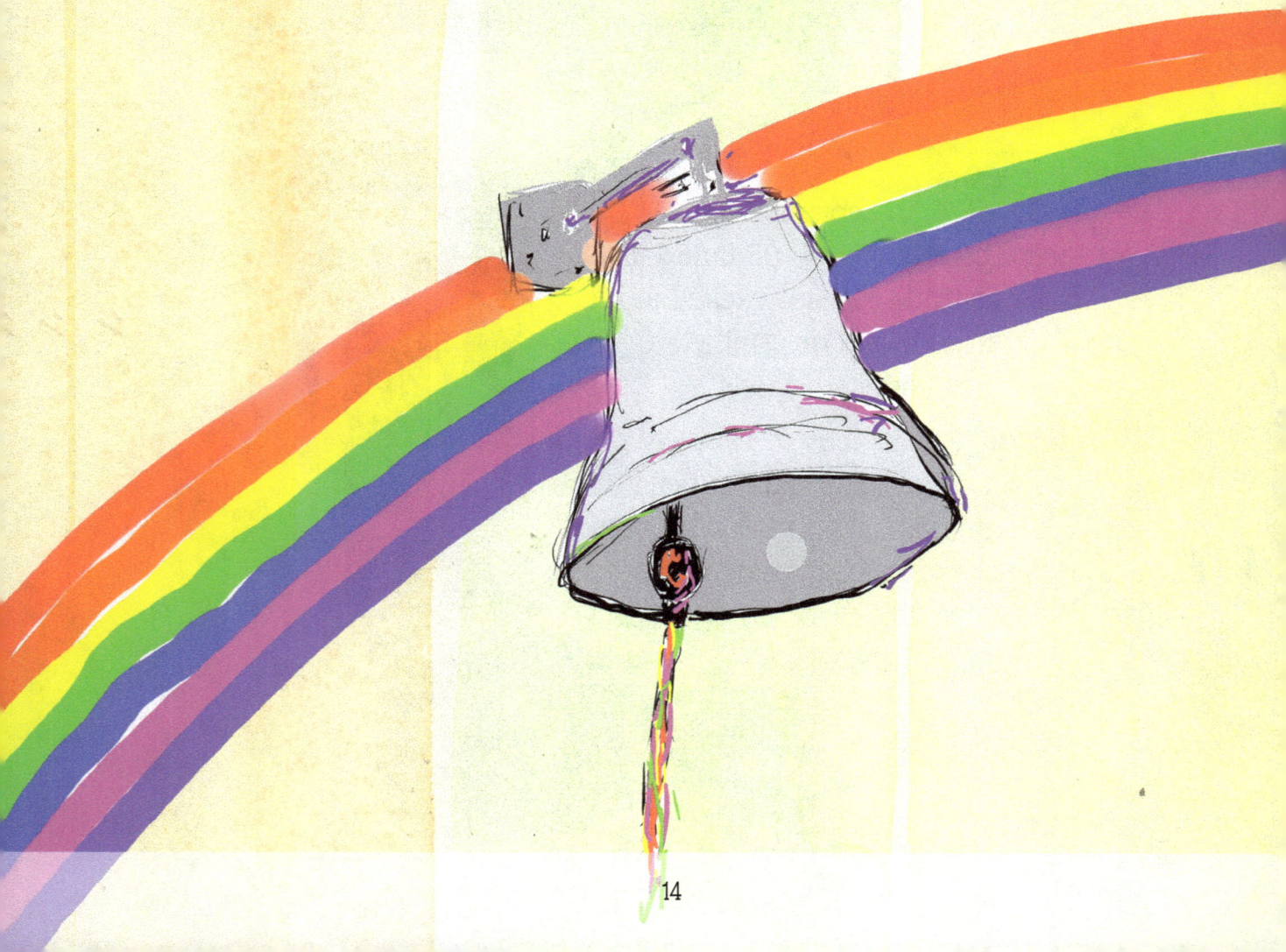

So, on my
last day, all of my family
came to the hospital.
We counted down my pump as it finished.
My family along with the doctors and
nurses lined up in the corridor,
and I gave a speech thanking
everyone.

Difficult roads often
lead to beautiful
Destinations...

'I am so thankful for all the nurses and doctors who helped me. I also thank my family for supporting me along the way', I said. 'And also, my nan who often stayed with me so mum and dad could have a rest. My aunty and cousins for visiting me and cheering me up, and my mum and dad for keeping me going. Oh, and of course, my little brother Tyler for being patient and understanding during my treatment'.

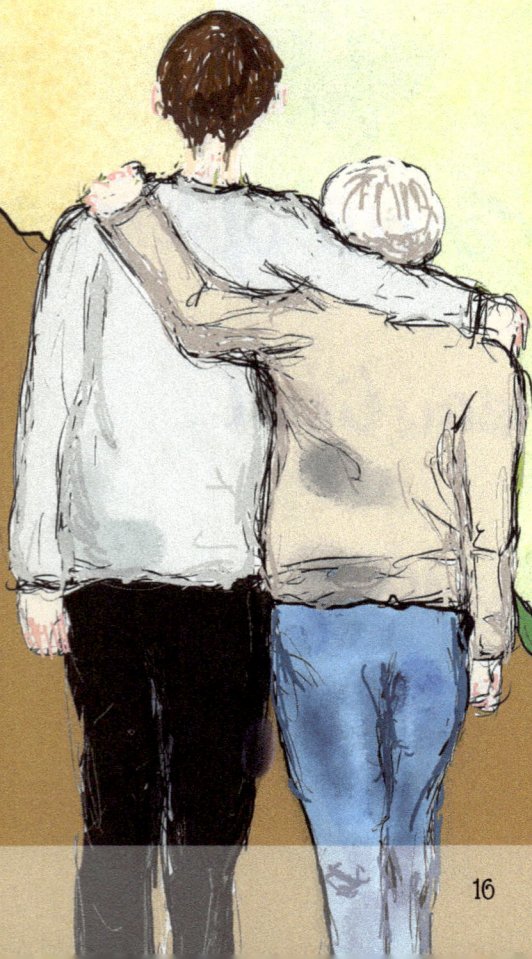

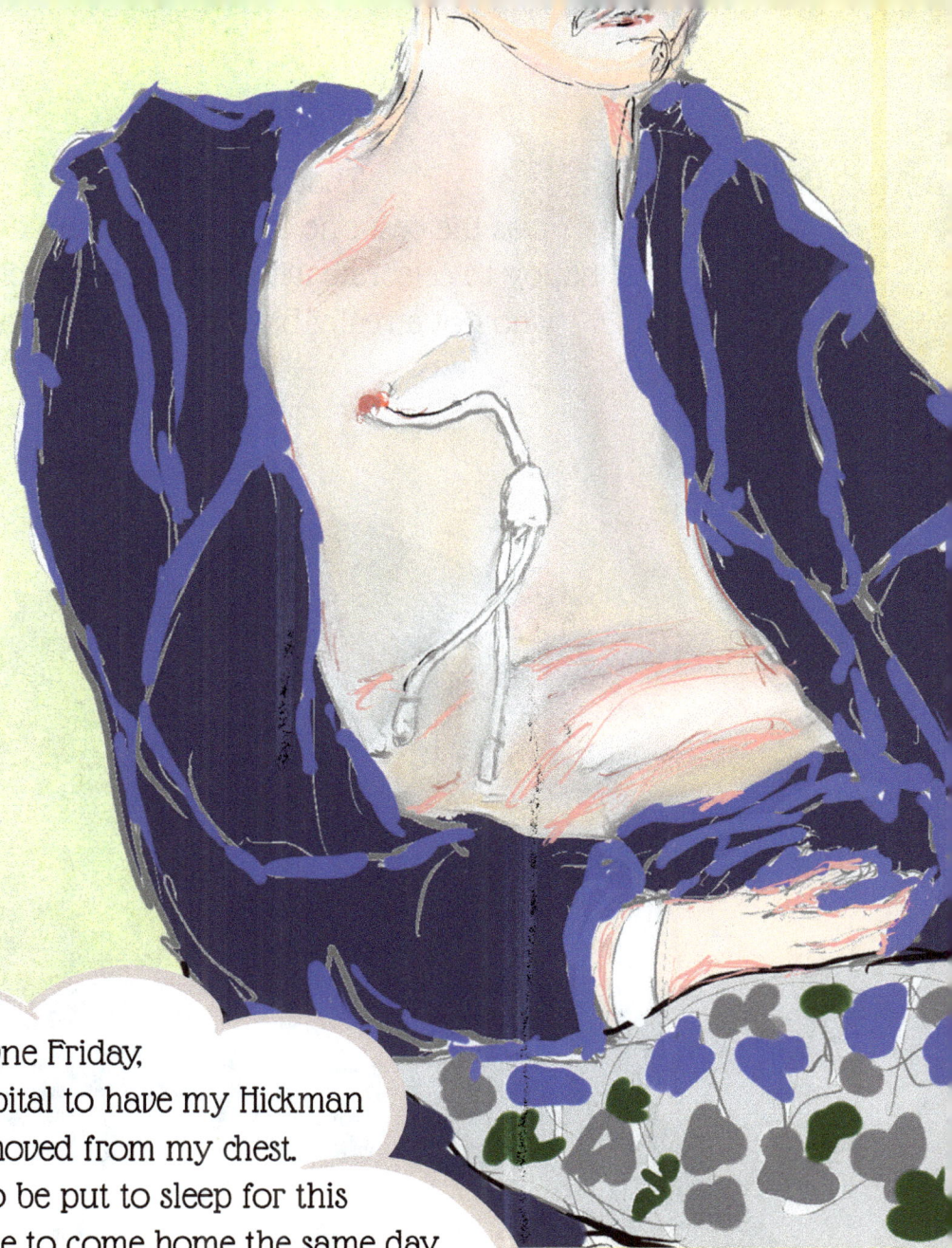

One Friday,
I went to hospital to have my Hickman
line removed from my chest.
I needed to be put to sleep for this
but would be able to come home the same day.
Oh, sorry, I forgot to tell you that a Hickman line is
a little tube the doctors put in your chest
for chemotherapy, we called it
the squiggly line.

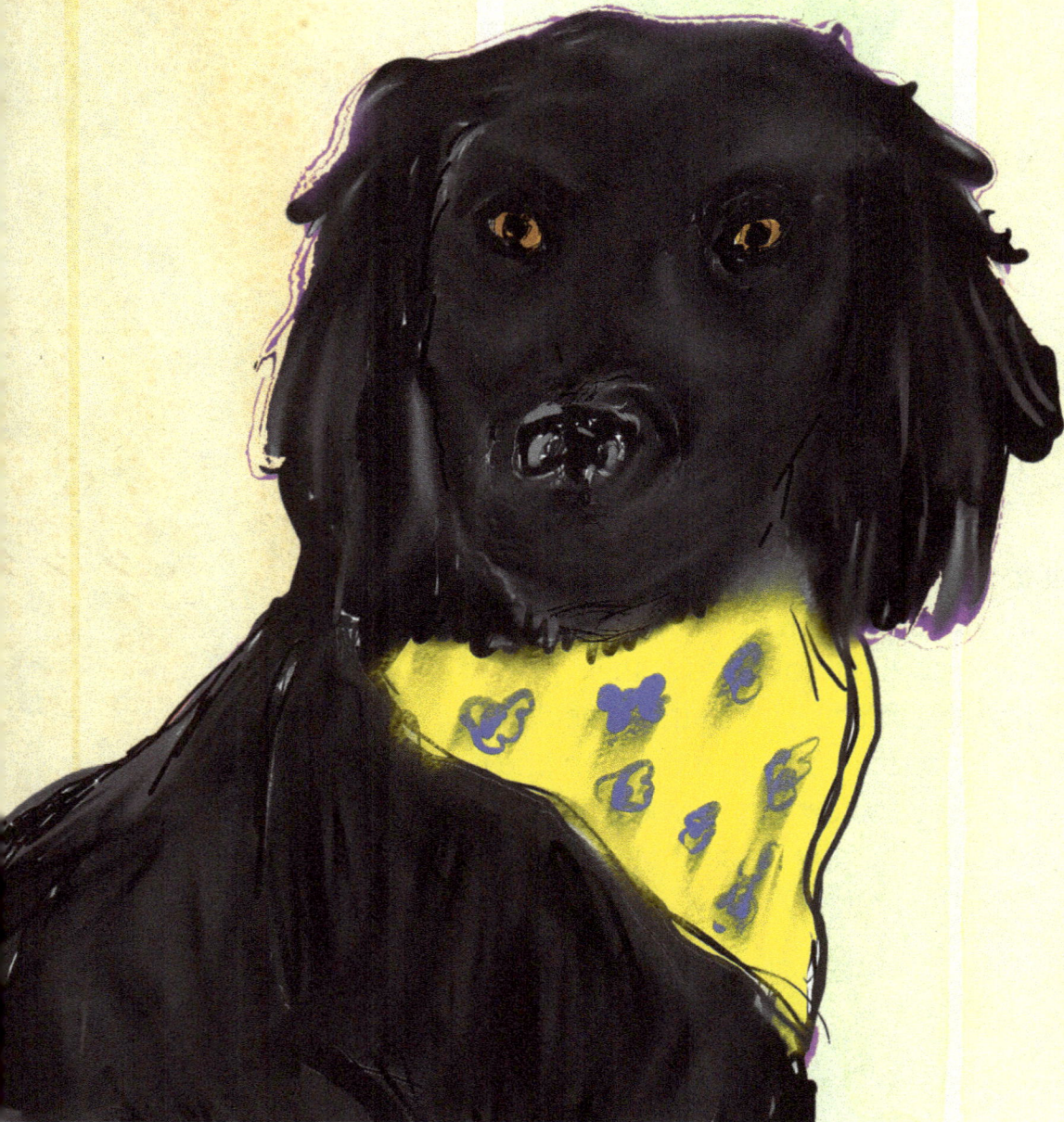

That Christmas
was the best one ever. I felt so thankful and
happy to celebrate with everyone, especially Buddy,
who got a really big, juicy bone for a present.

And guess what? There is something else, too!

In February, I got to have one of my biggest wishes come true thanks to the Make-A-Wish Foundation.

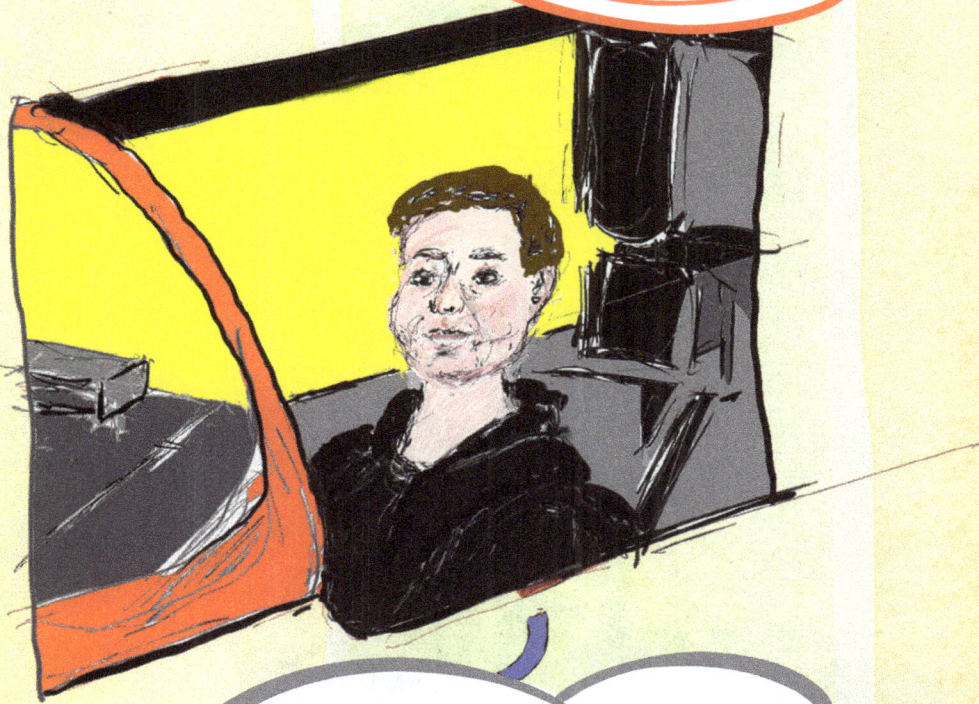

I knew Make-A-Wish was going to grant me a wish, and so I looked forward to it during my treatment and surgeries, and it made me so happy. They are a fantastic charity for kids going through what I went through. And guess who I got to meet? The Red Arrows! They're the Royal Air Force acrobatic team, pilots who do so many cool tricks! They are all so awesome, and it was amazing to get to meet them and see them fly their airplanes.

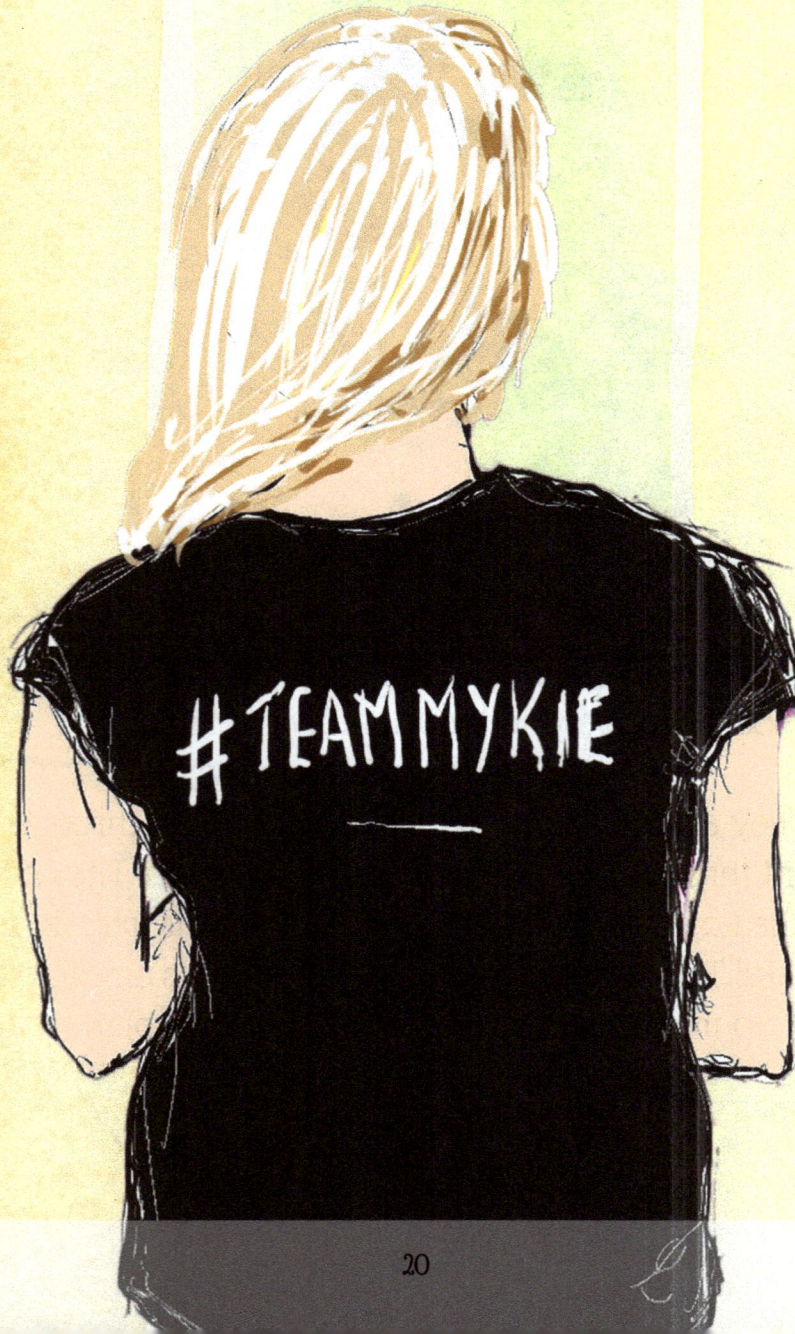

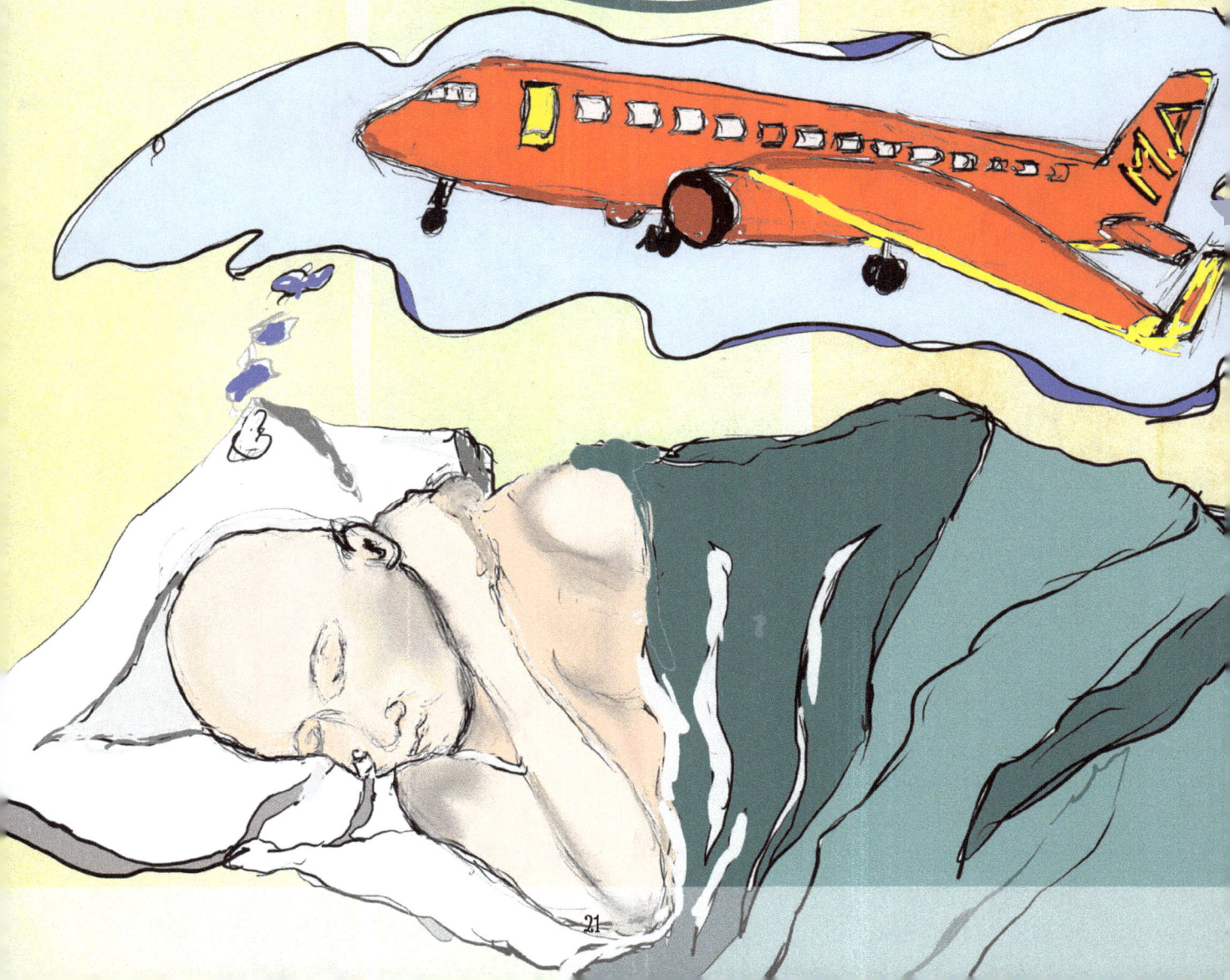

www.ingramcontent.com/pod-product-compliance
Lightning Source LLC
Chambersburg PA
CBHW080800300326
41914CB00055B/965